COLOUR
HEALING

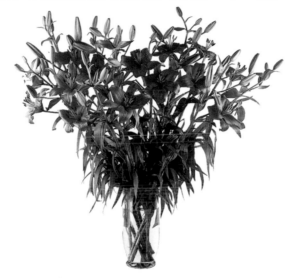

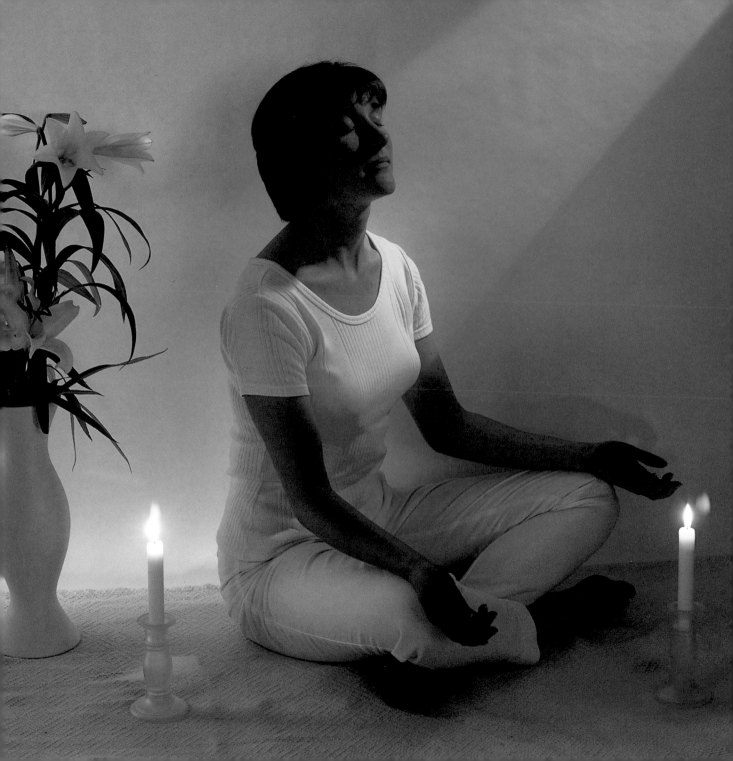

COLOUR
HEALING

A COMPLETE GUIDE TO RESTORING BALANCE AND HEALTH

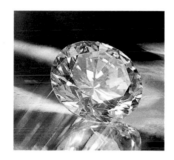

LILIAN VERNER-BONDS

LORENZ BOOKS

First published in 1999 by Lorenz Books

© Anness Publishing Limited 1999

Lorenz Books is an imprint of Anness Publishing Limited
Hermes House, 88-89 Blackfriars Road, London SE1 8HA

This edition distributed in Canada by Raincoast Books
8680 Cambie Street, Vancouver, British Columbia V6P 6M9

This edition published in the USA by Lorenz Books, Anness Publishing Inc.,
27 West 20th Street, New York, NY 10011; (800) 354-9657

ISBN 1 85967 898 X

A CIP catalogue record for this book is available from the British Library

Publisher: Joanna Lorenz, *Managing Editor:* Helen Sudell
Editorial Reader: Felicity Forster, *Production Controller:* Ben Worley
Designer: Nigel Partridge, *Photographer:* Don Last, *Illustrator:* Giovanni Pierce

Printd and bound in China

1 3 5 7 9 10 8 6 4 2

PUBLISHER'S NOTE
The reader should not regard the recommendations, ideas and techniques expressed and
described in this book as substitutes for the advice of a qualified medical practitioner or other
qualified professional. Any use to which the recommendations, ideas and techniques are put is at the
reader's sole discretion and risk.

CONTENTS

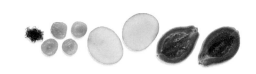

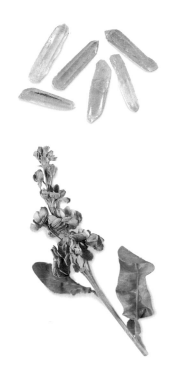

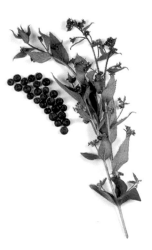

INTRODUCTION 6

THE PSYCHOLOGY OF COLOUR 12

COLOUR CONSCIOUSNESS 40

HEALING WITH COLOUR 50

INDEX AND ACKNOWLEDGEMENTS 64

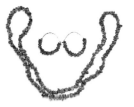

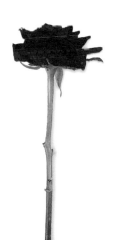

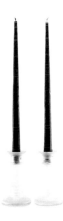

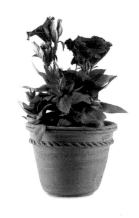

INTRODUCTION

WE ARE SWAMPED WITH COLOUR from the moment we are born. Indeed, we are born into a specific colour that stays with us for life. Colour is an aspect of everything we eat, drink, touch and are surrounded by. We use colours to describe our physical health, attitudes, emotions and even our spiritual or psychic experiences. Colour is an intimate part of our being, even though most of the time we take it for granted. However, it is impossible to be indifferent to colour. It affects every home environment, as well as those of factories, offices, schools and hospitals. Even the colours of your clothes reflect your personality and influence your mood, and colour has a practical bearing on all your personal relationships. Without light there is no life. If you put a plant in a dark cupboard, it will wither and die. Light is a natural requisite for growth and life, and, as living beings, we are continually reacting to the wide range of stimuli that we call light. From light come all the colours, each, as we will see in the following pages, with its own impact upon our systems.

Many of our healing needs can be met by the use of colour to bring about harmony and balance within the psyche and the body. The invisible vibrations of colour can either relax or stimulate us according to the colours chosen for healing. Even blind people can develop a sense of colour, by allowing the fingers to pick up the vibrational energy of different colours.

Looking closely at colour is a non-invasive way of discovering yourself. Its power is both transcendent and intuitive. Get to know what colour can do for you. Do not delay or neglect responding to this inner knowledge – colour can change your life.

◄ *Recharge your will and stamina by meditating on the ruby red petals of a rose.*

► *Discover more about your own nature by gazing into the pure colours of a rainbow bouquet.*

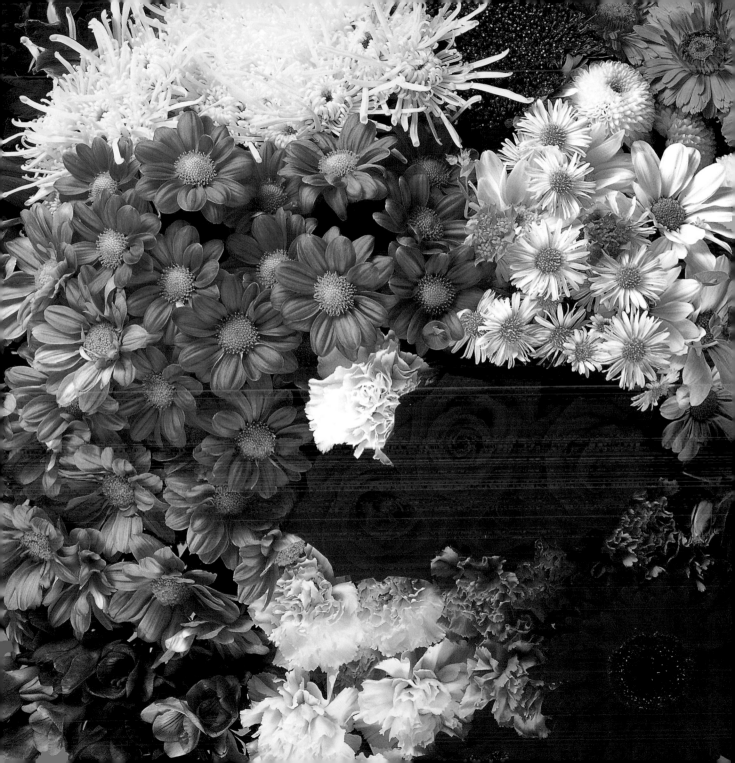

THE HISTORY OF HEALING WITH COLOUR

Ancient cultures worshipped the sun – whence all light, and therefore all colour, comes – and were aware of its healing powers. The therapeutic use of colour in the ancient world can be traced in the teachings attributed to the Egyptian god Thoth, known to the Greeks as Hermes. Following these teachings, Egyptian and Greek physicians – including Hippocrates, the father of Western medicine – used different coloured ointments and salves as remedies, and practised in treatment rooms painted in healing shades. In 1st-century Rome, the physician Aulus Cornelius Celsus wrote about the therapeutic use of colour, but with the coming of Christianity such ancient wisdoms came to be associated with pagan beliefs and were disallowed by the church.

The Arab physician Avicenna systematized the teachings of Hippocrates in the 9th century. He wrote about colour both as a symptom of disease and as treatment, suggesting, for example, that red would act as a stimulant on blood flow while yellow could reduce pain and inflammation.

Scientists and philosophers of the 18th century were concerned with the material world,

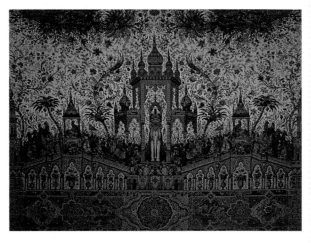

▲ *In many cultures, orange and red are associated with physical energy, creativity and life.*

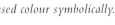

◄ *Medieval manuscripts used colour symbolically.*

and insisted on visible proof of scientific theories. Medicine focused on cures for physical ailments with advances in surgery and drugs, and less quantifiable healing techniques that dealt with spiritual and mental well-being were rejected.

Colour therapy re-emerged at the end of the 19th century. Edwin Babbitt, who published *The Principles of Light and Colour* in 1878, achieved world renown with his comprehensive theory, prescribing specific colours for a range of conditions.

Despite the medical establishment's continued scepticism, therapists in this century have developed the use of colour in psychological testing and

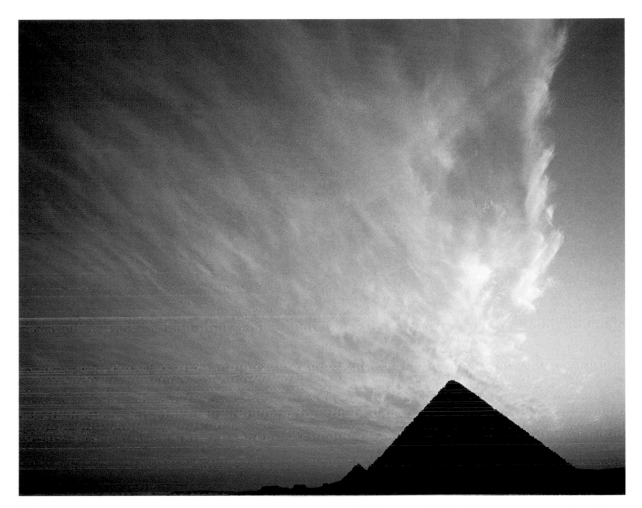

▲ *The Egyptians believed that the colour red had its strongest influence in the afternoon, and in the autumn.*

physical diagnosis. The Lüscher Colour Test was based on the theory that colours stimulate different parts of the autonomic nervous system, affecting metabolic rate and glandular secretions, and studies in the 1950s showed that yellow and red light raised blood pressure while blue light tended to lower it.

The use of blue light to treat neonatal jaundice is now common practice, and it has also been effective as pain relief in cases of rheumatoid arthritis.

LIGHT WAVES AND COLOUR

Light is a small portion of the electromagnetic spectrum, which also includes X-rays, ultraviolet and infrared light, microwaves and radio waves. The wave is the characteristic movement of all these types of energy, just like the waves on a body of water. Electromagnetic waves always travel in a straight line as they radiate out in all directions from their source.

The distance between two crests of a wave (the wavelength) determines which type of wave it is. Some wave-crests are over a metre apart – these are television and radio waves. Others are very close together – only billionths of a metre apart. These are gamma and cosmic rays. Around the middle of the spectrum is the tiny portion we experience as visible light.

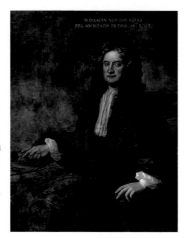

◀ *Most of today's understanding of colour has its roots in the work of Sir Isaac Newton.*

Within the visible spectrum, further gradations of wave-spacing produce different colours. The longest waves are at the red end of the spectrum, and the shortest at the purple end, with the other colours falling in between in order of their wavelengths. These pure colours are often referred to as "rays" by colour therapists. Just off either end of the spectrum visible to us are infrared and ultraviolet light, which are perceptible by other creatures such as snakes and honey bees.

Life on our planet has evolved to be able to perceive this narrow range of wavelengths. Other parts of the spectrum with long wavelengths (such as microwaves) or short wavelengths (such as X-rays) actually destroy living things. The sun, our local source of almost all of the electromagnetic spectrum, emits plenty of these long and short waves, but we are protected from them because our atmosphere screens them out at present – when we damage the atmosphere with pollution, we are ultimately harming ourselves.

◀ *A white beam shot through a prism registers all the colours of the electro-magnetic spectrum, from red to purple.*

▶ *The colour spectrum is the visible part of the electromagnetic spectrum.*

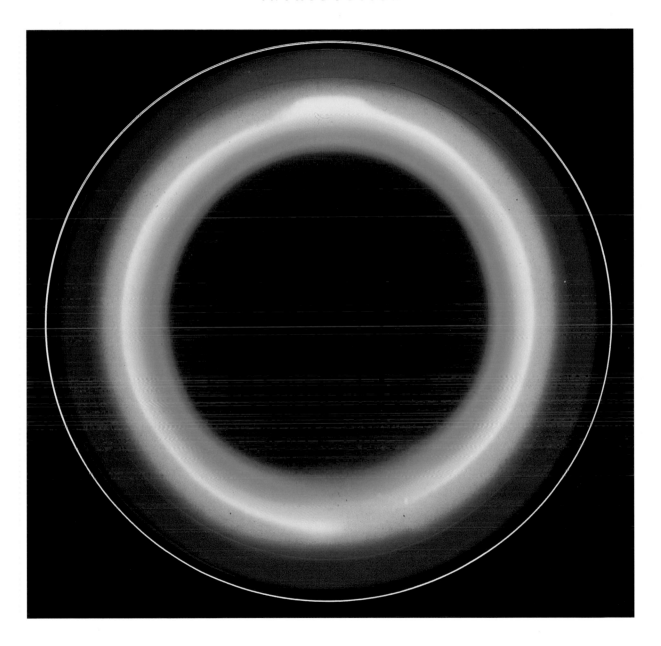

THE PSYCHOLOGY OF COLOUR

THE HUMAN BODY is intimately keyed to colour through its very evolution, and colour therapy is an important method of treatment. Colour affects your personality, whether because of cultural conditioning or your initial experience of a particular colour. If you have experienced a happy event in the past when you were wearing the colour blue, for example, it may remind you of special happenings.

We are influenced by the distinctive vibrations that each colour possesses. Each colour in the spectrum vibrates at its own rate and these vibrations correspond with the body's inner vibrations. Each part of the body resonates to a different colour. When we are ill or troubled we can use the appropriate colour to harmonize our vibrations and restore equilibrium.

There are psychological associations with each colour, and colours can be linked with moods. Reds, oranges and yellows are warm and expansive and give a feeling of energy, excitement

and joy. Blues, indigos and purples are calming and cooler. They quieten the temperament and induce relaxation. The psychology of colour is a language that you can learn, in the same way that you learn the alphabet in order to read and write. When you understand its basic meanings you can interpret what it reveals.

When you are well you may like most colours, but emotional and physical problems will tend to bring out preferences for different colours. Often you will be drawn to the colour you need, such as vigorous reds when you are exhausted. You will be naturally attracted to blues when you need some rest and healing. The over-excited would benefit from blues, but depression needs yellows and golds. This basic guide to colour will help you to check specifically what is happening in your system, and to choose the pertinent colour to correct the situation.

◀ *The colour energy of crystals has enormous potential for healing.*

▶ *The human psyche is wrapped in the colours of the rainbow.*

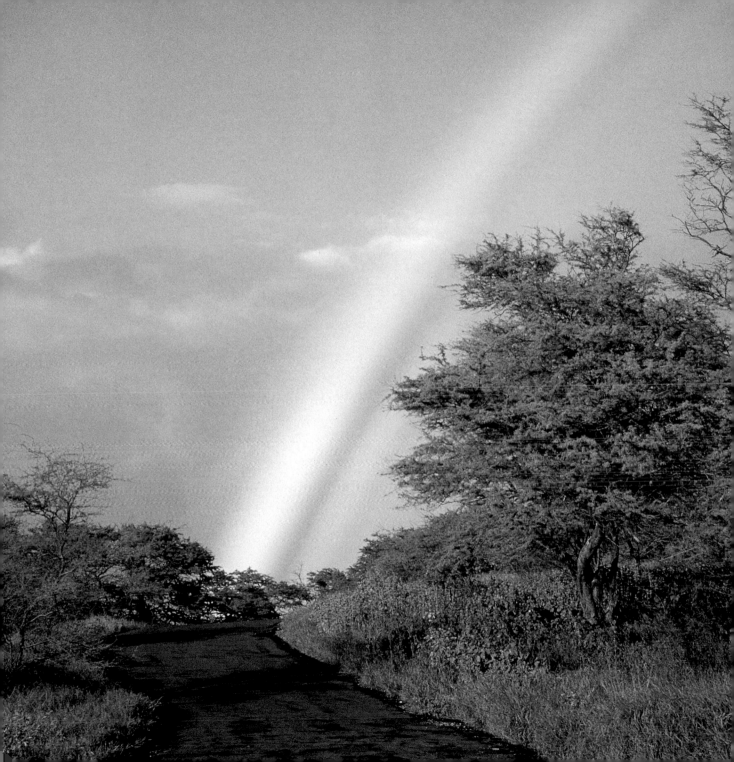

BRILLIANCE: THE RAY OF RAYS

Brilliance brings all rays of colour into perfect balance. Many people mistake brilliance for white, but brilliance is the light from which all colours spring. Brilliance is the clear light at the end of the tunnel that people recall after near-death experiences.

Brilliance itself is not a colour: it is the original or cosmic light. Brilliance represents the universal intelligence. It has the purity of the trinity of love, power and wisdom. Our local source of brilliance is the sun.

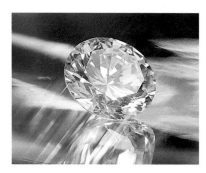

Without brilliance there can be no vision. Brilliance cuts directly through to the truth. It is the hard light that exposes all flaws and corruption. It contains the essence of all qualities, both

The transparent diamond in its clear brilliance sparkles with every colour of the rainbow.

positive and negative, sparkling in the brilliance of perfection. It clears the way for necessary actions. Brilliance clears any cloudiness in a person or colour. To recharge yourself at any time simply visualize pure brilliant light. When we say that someone is "brilliant", we are really acknowledging his or her purity of vision and action.

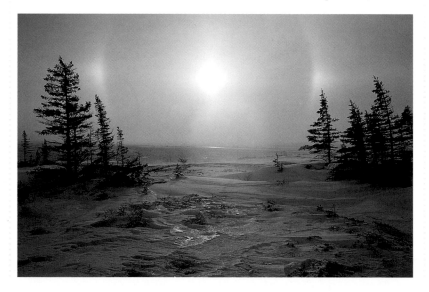

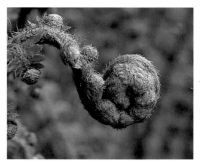

▲ *Brilliance makes all things grow. It is a state of perfection that exists within the cosmos.*

◀ *A burst of the sun's brilliance does wonders for the body and mind.*

14

BRILLIANCE AND PARTS OF THE BODY

Brilliance relates to the lymphatic system, and the tissues that filter out the debris from the body.

USING BRILLIANCE

Brilliance brings a ray of hope to your life when all seems lost. Brilliance brings change, whether you like it or not. It allows the delusions of your life to dissolve. Situations become clearer; you

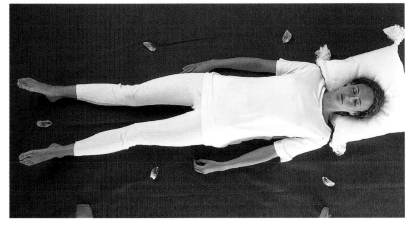

can wipe the slate clean and start again. It may bring about a move to a new home, a change of job, or a subtle inner transformation so that people recognize a new you. Old patterns fall away to be replaced with joy and an uplifting of the spirit.

Add a touch of brilliance to any colour and it will become brighter. Water is liquid brilliance: bathing in a waterfall is the equivalent of standing under a cascade of clear light. Or expose yourself to clear brilliance by taking a brief sunshine bath: you can renew yourself again and again.

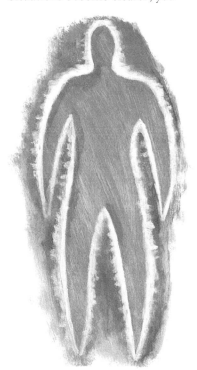

◀ *The glow of brilliance surrounds the whole body.*

▲ *This star-shaped placement of clear crystals around the body, known as the Seal of Solomon, increases clarity and quietens the mind, allowing brilliant insights to come into your consciousness.*

▼ *Brilliance captured in clear crystals encapsulates order, purity and clear thinking.*

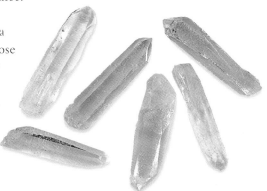

RED

Red is the spirit of physical life, full of power, fire and drive. It is courage and liberation, passion and excitement. Red has a burning desire to get somewhere, but tends to act without thinking. Red people are reformers and fighters, and at best are fine leaders. They are builders of great things from very little. They are explorers, with the energy of the life-force at their command. Pioneers – military and entrepreneurial – relate to red.

At its best, red will ensure a satisfying and passionate love life. Red at its worst is a tyrant or a brutal murderer, seeking advancement no matter who or what suffers.

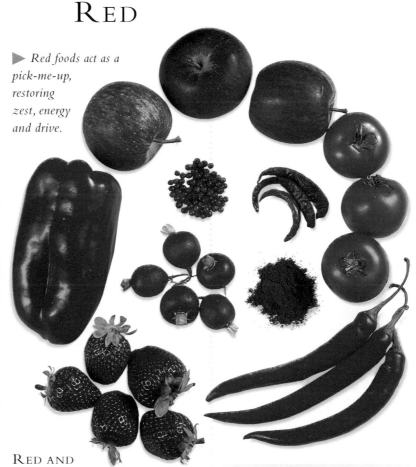

◀ *Red foods act as a pick-me-up, restoring zest, energy and drive.*

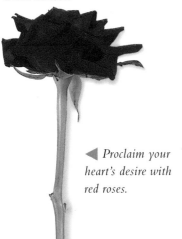

◀ *Proclaim your heart's desire with red roses.*

RED AND PARTS OF THE BODY
Red is associated primarily with the genitals and reproductive organs. The red glands are the gonads and the ovaries. Another area of red focus is the blood and circulation.

CAUTION
Do not use red lighting (chromotherapy) above the waist for heart conditions. Medical advice should be taken for any heart problem.

Red prompts the release of adrenalin into the bloodstream – hence its connection with aggression and fear. Problems that respond to red include a clogged circulation or irregularities in the blood supply, hardening of the arteries, infertility, exhaustion and anaemia.

USING RED

Red is a fiery force. It eliminates the unwanted and negativity. Red encourages the shy person to come out of themselves. It puts your life back into action. Red eases stiff muscles and joints, especially in the legs and feet. It is useful in cases of paralysis, especially when combined with physiotherapy (physical therapy). It acts as a tonic for anyone who catches colds or chills easily, and is good for a sluggish circulation.

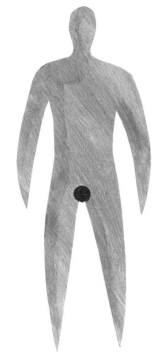

▲ *Red is the colour of the sexual organs.*

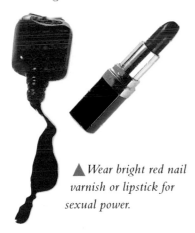

▲ *Wear bright red nail varnish or lipstick for sexual power.*

RED OPPOSITES
Expansion – Devastation

POSITIVE RED KEYWORDS
Chief • Resolute • Fighting • Vigorous • Diligent • Appreciative • Reviving

NEGATIVE RED KEYWORDS
Brutal • Lecherous • Prejudiced • Harsh • Bullying • Obstinate • Dishonourable

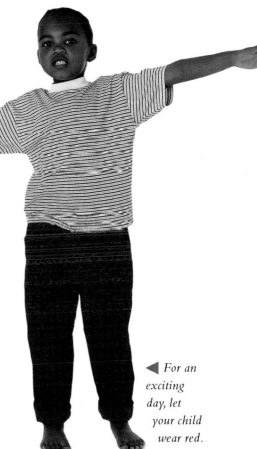

◀ *For an exciting day, let your child wear red.*

17

ORANGE

Orange is self-reliance and practical knowledge. In its role of assimilator, orange is the intestinal laboratory. It tests, then accepts or rejects. It has impetus, and is extremely persistent. But where red bullies, orange bides its time. Orange is genial, optimistic, tolerant, benign, warm-hearted. It is friendship, the life and soul of the party. The unkind practical joker is the negative orange.

Orange shatters; it breaks down barriers. Orange can eradicate. It brings up the energy of a past event that needs to be assimilated. Orange strength is subtle - it stimulates gently. It broadens life and is very purposeful. Orange moves on: it is the colour of divorce! Orange gives the courage to face the consequences. It accepts what is – and then changes it. Orange will not let sleeping dogs lie. It believes in the community. Orange people are usually skilled cooks or good at sport.

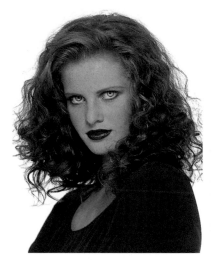

▲ *Bring changes into your life with the stimulation of orange: try the effect of a tawny hair colour.*

◀ *In the flower world, the orange marigold represents the doctor.*

▼ *This marmalade kitten's nine lives are bound to be lucky ones.*

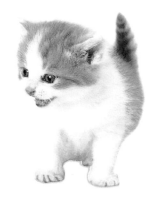

ORANGE OPPOSITES
Action – Indolence

POSITIVE ORANGE
KEYWORDS
Lavish • Tender • Unselfish •
Liberal • Brave • Genial •
Vital

NEGATIVE ORANGE
KEYWORDS
Arrogant • Gloomy •
Domineering •
Free-loading • Deceptive •
Vain

ORANGE AND
PARTS OF THE BODY
Orange is connected to the lower
back and lower intestines, the
abdomen and the kidneys. It
governs the adrenal glands and
our gut instincts.

USING ORANGE
Grief, bereavement and loss
respond well to treatment with
orange. Orange will
bring you
through the
shock of deep
outrage and will
give added strength
where it is needed to pull
through adversity. Orange

removes the inhibitions and
psychological paralysis that
occur when people are afraid of
moving forwards.

Asthma, bronchitis, epilepsy,
mental disorders, rheumatism,
torn ligaments and aching and
broken bones all respond to
treatment with orange. Orange
is also useful in alleviating
intestinal cramps.

▲ *Orange governs our gut instincts.*

▶ *Boost your dietary
assimilation with a
dash of orange.*

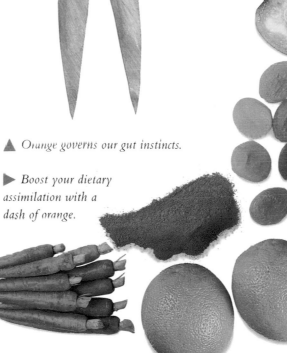

YELLOW

Yellow is the mind, precise and optimistic, clear and in control through the intellect. It is the colour of the scientist. It unravels and reveals, leaving no stone unturned. It focuses attention, loves new ideas and is flexible and adaptable. Yellow has no hesitation; it decides quickly and acts immediately.

Yellow smartens the reflexes. It is the great communicator: the journalist, the entertainer. It has no shortage of words. Yellow unifies and connects – a favourite pastime is networking. When something is revealed to yellow it immediately thinks of editing it for the public rather than feeling it for itself. Yellow is financial ambition – holding on to it may be more difficult. It

◀ Yellow clothes make you quick, alert and daring.

YELLOW OPPOSITES
Alertness – Evasion

POSITIVE YELLOW KEYWORDS
Fresh • Unprejudiced • Incisive • Fair • Speedy • Sharp • Honest

NEGATIVE YELLOW KEYWORDS
Cynical • Faithless • Preoccupied • Superficial • Hasty • Critical • Imprecise

is at the executive level of business and has the ability to get things done. Yellow despises pettiness. It has self-control, style and sophistication.

Yellow always broadcasts a feeling of well-being. People feel good around those under the yellow ray. They are sunny and willing, unless they are upset, when they can become acid and sharp-tongued.

Yellow is connected to the seat of self-confidence and self-esteem

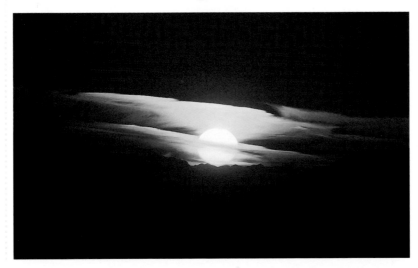

◀ Bask in the yellow sunset to help get your priorities right.

in the body. There is no fat on yellow – it is so quick that excess has no time to gather.

YELLOW AND PARTS OF THE BODY

Yellow is connected to the pancreas, solar plexus, liver, gall bladder, spleen, digestive system, middle stomach, the skin and the nervous system.

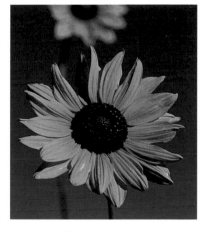

Yellow foods bring in the sunshine, releasing depression.

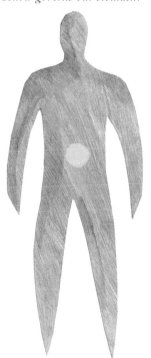

▼ *Yellow governs our stomach.*

USING YELLOW

Physically, yellow gets rid of toxins and stimulates the flow of gastric juices. Mentally, it clears away confusion and negative thinking. Emotionally, it boosts low self-esteem, lifts depression, and is particularly useful for fears and phobias.

Yellow is also good for menopausal flushes, menstrual difficulties and other hormonal problems. It sometimes helps to relieve the symptoms associated with diabetes, rheumatism and anorexia nervosa.

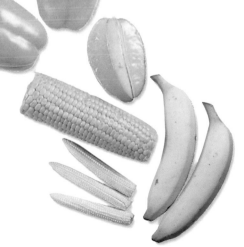

▲ *Sunflower yellow represents mental rigour and precise, clear thoughts.*

GREEN

Green is harmony; it stabilizes. Green is midway between red and purple: it is the bridge, the gateway in the spectrum – as the heart is in the body. The lesson of love needs to be learnt in order to cross green's bridge.

Green is idealistic, socially aware, helpful and selfless. Doctors and nurses are on the green ray. It is dependable and diplomatic. Green can see both sides but can be moralistic.

Green is clarity and understanding. It helps you to

GREEN OPPOSITES
Stable - Unstable

POSITIVE GREEN KEYWORDS
Discreet • Sensible • Fruitful • Benevolent • Tolerant • Talented

NEGATIVE GREEN KEYWORDS
Suspicious • Bitter • Unmindful • Greedy • Bland • Undependable • Disappointed

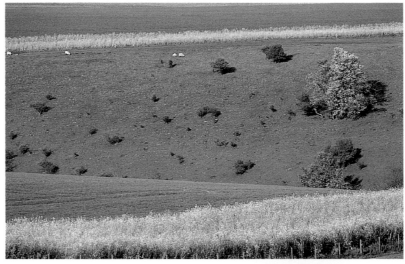

▲ *A walk in green fields will renew your connection with nature and restore your inner balance and harmony.*

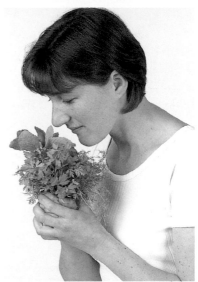

▶ *Nature's healing herbs incorporate the power of the colour green.*

do the best you can. Green is about finding one's niche. It is self-acceptance.

Green is prosperous, especially in business. Green is the "good life" and the love of collecting possessions. It is wanting the best. Positive green is the giver. It is

GREEN AND PARTS OF THE BODY

Green is connected to the thymus gland, heart, shoulders and chest, and the lower lungs.

USING GREEN

Green is made up of two primary colours: yellow and blue. Yellow brings clarity and blue brings insight. In combination, these two primaries aid memory. This makes green an important healing colour because most of our physical and mental illnesses result from events in the past.

Use green as a tonic. It is good for shock and fatigue. It helps biliousness, soothes headaches and is beneficial in cases of claustrophobia. It restores stability to anything malignant.

▼ *Green foods encourage detoxification and enhance physical stamina.*

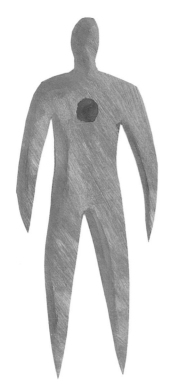

▲ *Green is the colour of the heart.*

generous and loves to share what it accumulates. It is a love of working outdoors.

Green can indicate difficulty in finding a settled way of life. There may be a conflict of ideas and emotions that causes commotion and upheaval. But with green's ability to discriminate and balance, this conflict can lead to correct judgement and action.

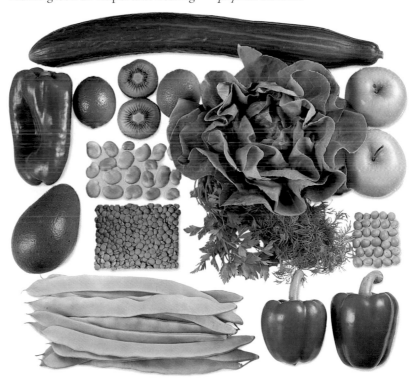

BLUE

Blue is the spirit of truth and the higher order of intelligence. The head and the heart speak directly through the blue throat.

Blue brings rest; it cools and calms; it slows down, and even retards growth. Blue is the tranquil spirit, the colour of contemplation. Its thinking is

▼ *Surround yourself with relaxing blues in the home.*

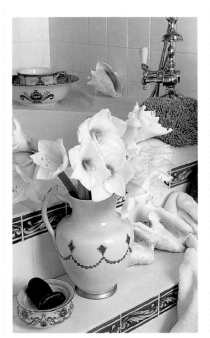

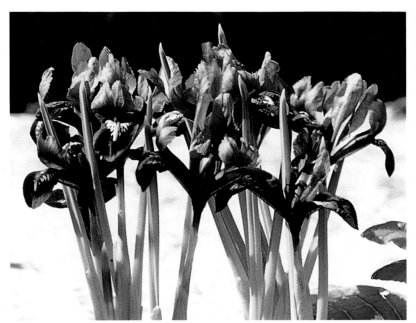

▲ *A bunch of blue flowers will help you to get into a contemplative mood.*

▼ *Use blue stones to promote a tranquil spirit.*

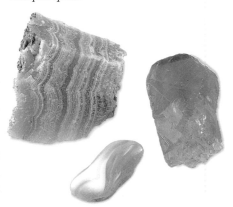

quiet and discriminating. "Still waters run deep" is a blue motto. Blue is peace with a purpose. Blue values integrity, honour and sincerity. It has a poised quality and will not easily draw attention to itself.

Although honesty is a blue keyword, its negative side is a master of manipulation, so skilled

BLUE OPPOSITES
Wisdom – Stupidity

POSITIVE BLUE
KEYWORDS
Serene • Virtuous • Sacred •
Reflective • Peaceful •
Harmonious • Faithful

NEGATIVE BLUE
KEYWORDS
Feeble • Emotionally
unbalanced • Malicious •
Egotistical • Unresponsive •
Dishonest • Ruthless

that you do not even know you have been manipulated. Blue does not like upsets or arguments – yet it often causes them. Blue always advises caution. It is highly inventive. Poetry, philosophy and writing are all blue professions.

BLUE AND
PARTS OF THE BODY
Blue is the throat area, upper lungs and arms, and the base of the skull; it relates to weight gain. The connected glands are the thyroid and parathyroids.

▶ *Blue governs our throat and our expression.*

USING BLUE
Because blue governs the throat, infections in this area are psychologically related to not speaking out. The blue personality hates arguments and often resorts to coughing and spluttering to avoid confrontation. The colour blue will help clear this by counteracting the deep internal

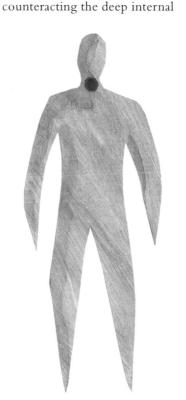

▶ *Blue foods promote tranquillity for jaded constitutions.*

terror of letting it all "spill out". A stiff neck, often representing the fear of moving forwards, can benefit from the application of blue. Children's ailments, such as teething, ear, throat and vocal problems can be treated with blue. It can also be used for incontinence.

Use a blue light bulb to flood the sickroom with blue light – it cools and calms. It is particularly useful in reducing fevers, and for the terminally ill.

INDIGO

Indigo has force and power. It transmutes and purifies. It unravels the unknown; it can see more than is apparent.

There is no in-between for indigo: it is all or nothing. Indigo is very conscious of the rungs of the ladder. To be out of step is a fate worse than death for indigo.

Indigo aspires to be a spiritual master: it is the inspired preacher and writer. Indigo can reconcile science and religion. But blind devotion is an indigo failing. Negative indigo is the believer who has become a fanatic. All addictions relate to negative indigo. Indigo knows when to move and when to hold fast. It constantly pushes you into reviewing your life. As structure is an indigo aspect, it promotes justice and peace. Lawyers and actors relate to indigo.

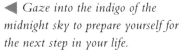 *Gaze into the indigo of the midnight sky to prepare yourself for the next step in your life.*

Meditate with indigo candles to transmute and purify your life.

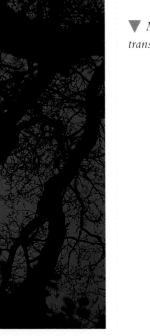

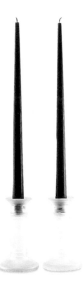

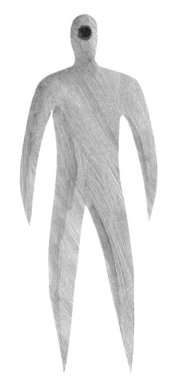

▲ *Indigo represents the skeleton*

INDIGO AND PARTS OF THE BODY

Indigo represents our bone structure, especially the backbone, and also the pituitary gland, the lower brain, eyes and sinuses.

USING INDIGO

Indigo is the strongest painkiller in the spectrum. It can clear up bacteria and the results of air, water and food pollution.

Indigo is good for acute sinus problems, which psychologically are often uncried tears from childhood. Use it for chest complaints, bronchitis, asthma, and for the treatment of lumbago and sciatica, migraine, eczema and inflammations. It helps to bring down high blood pressure and is particularly effective for an over-active thyroid. It is helpful in the control of diarrhoea and is the best antidote for insomnia. It aids kidney complaints and disperses growths, tumours and lumps of any kind. Emotionally, it can help to cure deep hurt.

INDIGO OPPOSITES
Devout – Faithless

POSITIVE INDIGO
KEYWORDS
Discerning • Organized •
Optimistic • Tenacious •
Pure • Compliant

NEGATIVE INDIGO
KEYWORDS
Immoderate • Authoritarian •
Submissive • Puritanical •
Obsessed • False

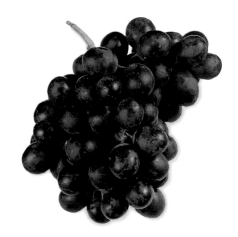

▲ *Put some structure back into your life with indigo foods and experience its steadfast energy.*

▼ *Hold an indigo crystal to unravel the unknown.*

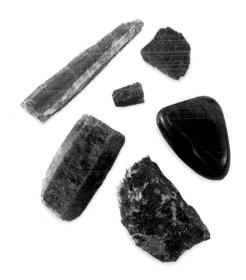

PURPLE

Purple is the royal ray, the ruler, the spiritual master. It is also the protector and the spirit of mercy. Purple is the aristocracy of the spirit; it strives for enlightened perfection. Purple is the visionary; it works with the highest levels of thought, seeing and hearing without using the physical senses. Purple uses its psychic perception on an everyday basis.

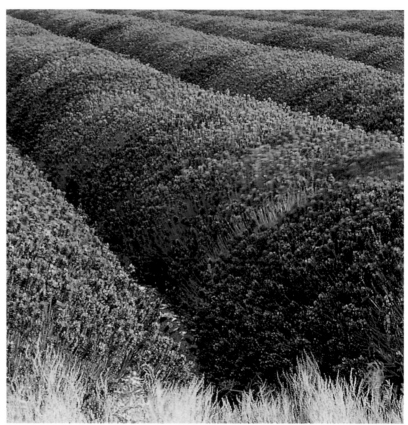

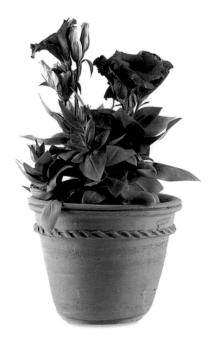

▲ *Amethyst is the great protector. Look out on a lavender field to feel its comforting cloak of security.*

◄ *Place purple flowers near you when you are working, to relieve eyestrain.*

CAUTION
Purple light should never be directed on to the face, but applied only to the back of the head.

Purple comes to understand that the price it must pay for its royal attributes is sacrifice. Humility is a key aspect. But it can sacrifice itself for the benefit of all without being a victim or a martyr. Negative purple can be belligerent and treacherous.

Purple is the great teacher who realizes that the pupil has to understand – facts alone are not

▼ *Purple is the colour of the brain.*

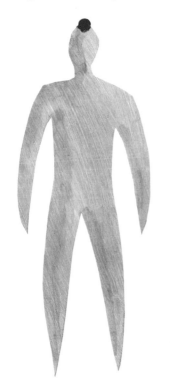

PURPLE OPPOSITES
Serenity – Hostility

POSITIVE PURPLE KEYWORDS
Magisterial • Altruistic • Noble • Personal • Artistic • Boundless • Mystic

NEGATIVE PURPLE KEYWORDS
Merciless • Spiritually haughty • Self-important • Depraved • Snobbish • Dictatorial

enough. Clergymen, musicians and painters all work with the colour purple.

PURPLE AND PARTS OF THE BODY
Physically, purple represents the top of the head – the crown, the brain and the scalp – as well as the pineal gland.

USING PURPLE
Purple is a colour to be used sparingly. It is a "heavy" colour, and long exposures to purple may be depressing. It can reveal deep-rooted depression and even suicidal tendencies.

▼ *Purple foods will help put you in the right mood to face conflicts in your life.*

It is a useful colour, good for any kind of internal inflammation and for subduing palpitations of the heart. Purple is a good colour for head problems or any irritation of the scalp. The immune system and jangled nerves can also benefit from purple. It is not recommended for use with children, whether in clothing or lighting; if it is used with children, exposure times should be kept very short or it could be introduced in lighter shades first.

Should you suffer from an overload of purple, the antidote is exposure to gold – gold lighting, decor or clothes.

29

BLACK

Black is the colour of the person who keeps control by not giving information to others. Black indicates that something is lying dormant or buried. It is connected to philosophical thoughts and ideals.

Someone wearing black continuously may be saying that there is something absent from his or her life. Negative black believes that all is ended, there is nothing to look forward to. It is afraid of what is coming next.

◀ *Dressing in black says: "I'm young, I'm ready and I'm totally in control."*

▶ *Wearing black jewellery will announce "I have hidden potential."*

But at the heart of black is discipline: this brings about freedom, which is wonderfully liberating. Any cause that gives genuine support and works toward the light is working with the magic of black. Black can complete the incomplete. The mystic arts relate to black.

BLACK AND PARTS OF THE BODY
There are no parts of the body specifically connected to black except when seen on X-rays or in the aura as disease.

USING BLACK
Use black in a positive way to encourage self-discipline. To break the stagnation of black, introduce colours. Encourage the person to reach out.

◀ *A black feather represents respect for the old.*

BLACK OPPOSITES
Abundance – Nothingness

POSITIVE BLACK KEYWORDS
Beneficially strong •
Creative • Idealistic •
Secretly wealthy

NEGATIVE BLACK KEYWORDS
Destructively strong •
Troublesome • Superior •
Despairing • Constrained

▼ *Black foods heighten your awareness of the magic within you.*

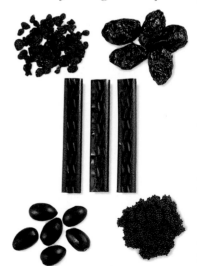

WHITE

White is next to the cosmic intelligence of brilliance, a denser brilliance. White has just stepped down from the ultimate purity of brilliance. Its fundamental quality is that all colours are equal in white. White has supreme faith, which it derives from reason. It conjures up hope, but on the negative side white is its own worst enemy.

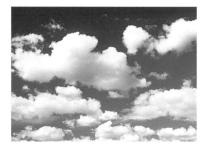

▲ *Gazing into white clouds creates simplicity and a wonderful feeling of transcendental perfection.*

▼ *Bridal white symbolizes purity in the human form.*

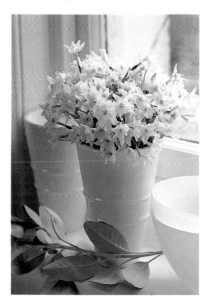

White travels light, so it's drawn to professions that are streamlined and precise. The civil service, banking and ergonomics suit it well.

WHITE AND PARTS OF THE BODY
The eyeball is connected to white: its shades of whiteness are used in diagnosis.

USING WHITE
As white contains equal amounts of all the colours, it does not distinguish one organ from another. Wear it as a tonic to top up the colours in your body's system.

WHITE OPPOSITES
Unspoiled – Dirty

POSITIVE WHITE KEYWORDS
Unsullied • Comprehensive • Benevolent • Truthful • Concordant

NEGATIVE WHITE KEYWORDS
Secluded • Barren • Harsh • Rigid • Unsuccessful

▼ *White foods help to clear the lymphatic system of debris.*

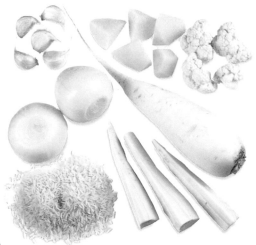

GOLD

Gold is purity. Gold means "I am". It does not seek, it has already found. It is the soul's experience of all that is past. Gold has access to knowledge and – most important – to knowledge of the self. It is forgiveness and letting go of the past out of a deeper understanding. It expands the power of love because it trusts completely.

Negative gold will blow its own trumpet. Gold's conceit is that of privilege and belief in itself as inherently more worthy than others.

True gold is a belief in honour among men. Gold is extremely gracious. It has the gift to release, but it knows what is needed. Gold is related to the wise old sage.

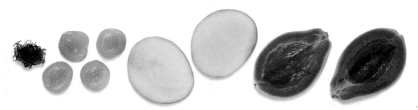

▼ *Golden foods symbolize trust, which allows success to follow.*

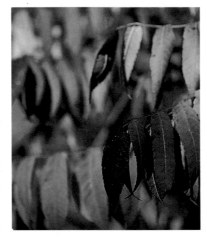

▲ *Golden berries and leaves have the fruitfulness of maturity.*

GOLD AND PARTS OF THE BODY

No parts of the body connect with gold, an offshoot of yellow. It can be seen in auras, however.

USING GOLD

Gold is very beneficial for both physical and psychological depressions – it is uplifting. It dissipates suicidal tendencies. It is good for any kind of digestive irregularity, irritable bowel syndrome, rheumatism and an underactive thyroid. Gold is beneficial for the treatment of scars and scar tissue.

▶ *Gold jewellery represents the well-heeled; it is naturally associated with money and wealth.*

GOLD OPPOSITES
Faith – Doubt

POSITIVE GOLD KEYWORDS
Mature • Enlightened •
Abundant • Lenient •
Achieving

NEGATIVE GOLD KEYWORDS
Cynical • Mistrusting •
Obstructive • Sullen •
Misfitting

32

SILVER

Silver is the thread of cosmic intelligence. An invisible silver cord is said to attach us to "the other side". It stills the emotions and is the great natural emotional tranquillizer. Silver illuminates and pierces; it lights up the path. It penetrates and lays bare. The silvered mirror reflects: it can reveal that a person is full of illusion and living a life that doesn't exist.

Negative silver shows up in relationships in which there is no substance, just delusion. People who fall in love with stars of the

SILVER OPPOSITES
Increasing – Decreasing

POSITIVE SILVER KEYWORDS
Revealing • Contemplative • Impartial • Astute • Flowing

NEGATIVE SILVER KEYWORDS
Deceitful • Disconnected • Slippery • Inauthentic

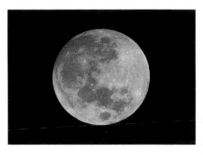

▲ *The silvery moon has the two faces of sadness and romance. It is also the greatest natural tranquillizer – it stills the emotions.*

▼ *Surround a favourite image with the endurance of a silver-coloured frame.*

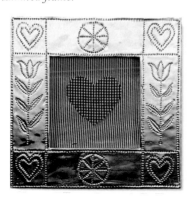

silver screen are under the negative of silver. Professions that create make believe work under silver's influence.

Silver resolves disputes. It takes an unbiased stand.

SILVER AND PARTS OF THE BODY

There are no body parts specifically connected to silver. The feminine dimension of the self is silver, whether it resides in a male or female body.

▶ *Use silver cutlery for an important lunch to ensure unbiased discussions.*

USING SILVER

Silver is good for calming the nerves as well as the hormones. It harmonizes and brings about a fluid state of consciousness. Bathe in the moonlight to restore your equilibrium.

TURQUOISE

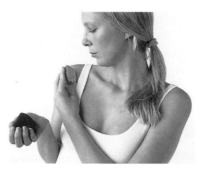

▲ *The stillness of a turquoise stone calms the panic that follows emotional shock.*

Turquoise is single-minded and looks to itself first. It is the colour that says: "Stand still! What do I think? What do I need?" Turquoise says what it feels rather than what is appropriate. Its basic motivation in life is personal relationships. Negative turquoise can be deceived about itself. It

◀ *A turquoise silk scarf will allow you to speak up for yourself in your relationships.*

can be an emotional manipulator. The antique business is well suited to turquoise, as is working with animals. Turquoise is good at sharing as it hates to be alone. It just loves family life.

▼ *Turquoise jewellery is the greatest healer for affairs of the heart.*

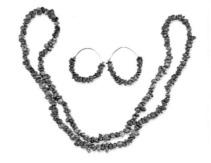

TURQUOISE AND PARTS OF THE BODY
Turquoise is connected to the throat and chest.

USING TURQUOISE
Turquoise feeds the central nervous system and soothes the throat and chest. Turquoise also encourages self-questioning and coming to know what you want. It helps you to get on with life. Turquoise can help to dispel emotional shock.

▼ *Step into a turquoise sea to restore peace within yourself.*

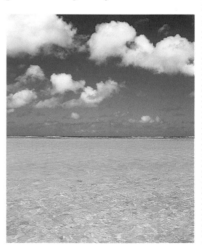

TURQUOISE OPPOSITES
Autonomy – Egotism

POSITIVE TURQUOISE KEYWORDS
Calm • Introspective • Self-reliant • Self-possessed

NEGATIVE TURQUOISE KEYWORDS
Reserved • Indecisive • Undependable • Boastful • Narcissistic

GREY

Grey is the bridge between black and white, where innocence and ignorance meet. Grey at its best is optimistic, and knows that the best is yet to come. At its weakest, it believes it cannot have it today. It might get it tomorrow… but tomorrow never comes.

Negative grey is conventional to the point of narrow-mindedness. It is the shade of suffering and poverty.

Grey offers a helping hand. It helps one break free the chains that bind. Grey usually does the jobs that no one else wants to do.

GREY OPPOSITES
Black – White

POSITIVE GREY KEYWORDS
Well-versed • Sane • Authentic • Reputable • Spartan

NEGATIVE GREY KEYWORDS
Destitute • Carping • Dispirited • Ill • Miserable • Depressed

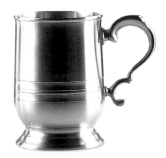

▲ *The bright grey of pewter opens one up to receive grace and understanding.*

GREY AND PARTS OF THE BODY
There are no body parts connected specifically to grey, but when grey appears it represents breakdown.

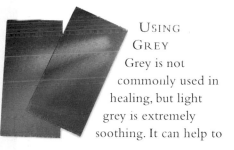

USING GREY
Grey is not commonly used in healing, but light grey is extremely soothing. It can help to

▲ *Slate-grey is the colour of austerity. There is a belief in grey that there is never going to be enough.*

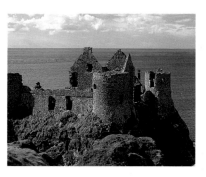

▲ *Grey can be divine in its destruction, because it makes way for renewal.*

restore sanity. When the skin and nails have a grey tint, it is an indicator of congestion somewhere in the body.

▼ *Grey chains represent persistence and endurance.*

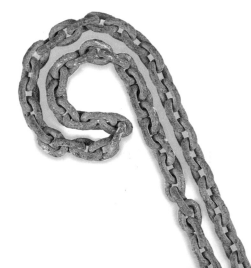

SHADES AND TINTS

When we talk about colour we usually refer to the hue, which indicates a single colour such as green, blue or red. However, each colour has many facets, and appears in many different guises.

Colours may be experienced as light or dark, bright or dull; touches of other colours in the spectrum result in many variations of tone within each colour.

▼ *All tints have a proportion of white in them, and all shades have black.*

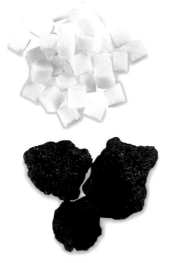

◀ *Pink is constant affection, loving and forgiving.*

All tones of a colour share that colour's underlying qualities, but their psychological meanings are modified according to whether they are a higher (tint) or lower (shade) tone of the colour. For instance, scarlet, crimson and flame are the most active of the reds. Reds with a touch of brown – russet and maroon – are more subdued and cautious in character. Pinks, which are tints of red, are much lighter and gentler than the basic colour.

Colour therapists work with the seven colours of the spectrum together with their shades and tints. Pale

▶ *Emerald green is connected to wealth and abundance.*

▶ *Pale blue is the soul searching for maturity.*

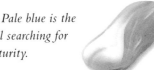

colours – tints – have more white in them, which makes them stronger for healing. For instance, pale pink is more powerful than the basic hue of red because of the abundance of white it contains. Shades of a colour are darker, with the basic hue mixed with black.

Generally speaking, the tints of any colour are considered positive and the shades negative. But the negative can be useful too, because it can alert us to problems that we may need to identify and address.

RED
MAROON: Subdued and cautious; deeply thoughtful; overcomes adversity.
MAGENTA: Spiritually uplifting; the great improver and arbiter.
CRIMSON: Does not believe in strife; strong but kind; tenacity and freedom.

▲ *The shade violet is always striving for spiritual awareness.*

SCARLET: Love of life; willingness.
PINK: Comforting and mollifying; ripeness; affection.

ORANGE
DARK ORANGE: Undermining; the gambler; the loser.
AMBER: Gives confidence and supports self-confidence.
PEACH: Helps communication; impeccable behaviour.

YELLOW
DARK YELLOW: Low self-esteem; gloomy; the grumbler.
LEMON YELLOW: Orderly; brittle; the misfit; astute.
CITRINE YELLOW: Capricious; superficial.

PRIMROSE YELLOW: Supersensitive; searching.
CREAM: Expansion of space; reassurance; slackness.

GREEN
DARK GREEN: Possessiveness; blindness to another's needs; remorse or resentment.
OLIVE GREEN: Self-deception; bitterness; endurance; mercy.
EMERALD GREEN: Material affluence; easy-going nature; abundance.
JADE GREEN: Generosity of spirit; balanced, natural wisdom.
PALE GREEN: Fresh starts; immaturity; inability to make up one's mind; unhappy childhood.

BLUE
DARK BLUE: Focused; Just; a worrier; repressed.
AZURE BLUE: Supreme happiness; contentment with a purpose;

▼ *The indigo shade has the power to see what cannot be seen.*

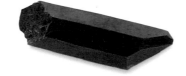

◄ *Peach, a tint of orange, puts forth the quality of gentle persuasion.*

release from bondage and tyranny.
SKY BLUE: Calm, constant love; ability to overcome all obstacles.
PALE BLUE: Uplifting; ambitious; a giver; determined to succeed.

INDIGO
DARK INDIGO: Always waiting in the wings; the dawn never comes. (Indigo does not have a tint.)

PURPLE
DEEP PURPLE: Arrogance; corrupt power; delusion; ruthlessness.
VIOLET: Adores to revere; a rebuilder of hope; intuition; sense of destiny.
AMETHYST: Mystical connections; idealism; protects the vulnerable.
MAUVE: Makes the right choices; aristocratic; dynastic.
PLUM: Old-fashioned; pompous; full of false pride; boring.
LAVENDER: Perceptive and fragile; elusive; aesthetic.
LILAC: A bright personality; vanity; glamour; romance; adolescence.

HIDDEN COLOURS

When working with colour it is important to be aware of what are termed hidden colours, particularly when using colours for healing. Orange, for instance, is made up of the hidden colours of red and yellow. The eye will see orange but the body will also experience the red and yellow vibrations that are within the orange. Therefore, when working with orange for healing, look for the psychological aspects that relate to red and yellow as well as to orange.

The colour green has its own healing meaning, plus the yellow and blue that make up green. Similarly, purple has red and blue within it, so remember to evaluate these colours also. Grey, of course, consists of the hidden colours black and white.

All these hidden colours are important for their psychological meanings and are not to be confused with the pigments artists use for painting.

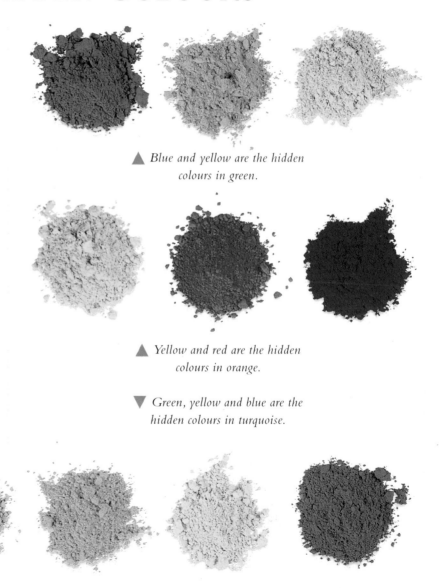

▲ *Blue and yellow are the hidden colours in green.*

▲ *Yellow and red are the hidden colours in orange.*

▼ *Green, yellow and blue are the hidden colours in turquoise.*

COMPLEMENTARY COLOURS

Every colour of the spectrum has an opposite colour that complements it. This is particularly helpful for healing and can be used in everyday life. It enables you to pinpoint instantly the appropriate colour for support and help.

For example, if you feel extremely irritable and furious at someone's behaviour, at that moment you will be reacting to an overload of red vibration within your system. To counteract this, just think of blue, put on some blue clothing or gaze at a blue object. Continue to do this until you

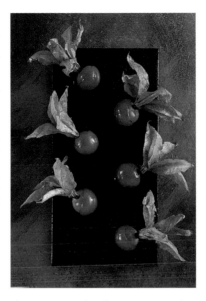

▲ *Orange and indigo support each other when used for healing.*

◀ *Red is the colour of efficiency and activity, while blue calms and stills the mind and body.*

feel the anger pass. Or you may find yourself in a room with yellow decor that you find disturbing. Rather than leave, close your eyes and conjure up the colour purple, the complementary of yellow, to dispel the vibration of the yellow.

The complementary colour of red is blue, that of orange is indigo and yellow's is purple. Green, the middle colour of the rainbow, has magenta, which is made up of red and blue, as its complementary. This index can also be of use when you are using a lamp with coloured slides for healing. For instance, use a blue slide to relieve the red of irritability, or vice versa – use a red slide to pull you out of the blues you find yourself in.

If you are ever in doubt about a colour, or have a feeling that too much colour has been used, just flood yourself with green – if you are using a lamp – or visualize it. Green acts as a neutralizer, returning balance and order to any situation.

▼ *Use green to balance an overabundance of white.*

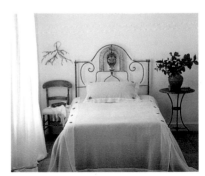

COLOUR CONSCIOUSNESS

IT HAS BEEN OBSERVED that the absence of light can cause a person to suffer both in body and mind. So it is important when creating a home environment that you take into consideration the sunlight that penetrates your rooms. Exposing the occupants to as much sunlight as possible increases their chances of remaining healthy. Although it is unwise to sit exposed to the direct rays of the sun unprotected, it is important that the glow from the sun's beams is received into your psyche. As a radical figure in the development of health care, Florence Nightingale was well aware of the purifying effect of sunlight. Allowing sunlight to flood into dark corners rids any room of its staleness and kills some bacteria. It also lifts the spirits. We reach out towards the light and withdraw from its absence.

Colour is a sensation. It enriches the world and our understanding of it, and we use it as a code. A knight of old would give his lady his personal colours to wear before he went into battle. Colour helps us to determine when fruit and vegetables are ripe. Our skin changes colour with shock, shyness or excitement. Too much yellow light can cause arguments between people, and blue light can quieten them. Colour enriches our lives, whether it is red for danger and green for go, a purple and gold sunset, or a beautiful rainbow.

Colour leads into all realms of life on earth and in the universe. There is a mystery about colour that bewitches us. It is there for us to use, and there is no better way to use it than by harnessing its strength and benefits to enhance our homes and environment.

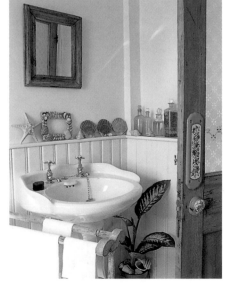

◀ *Relaxing in a green bathroom will soothe headaches and act as a general tonic to help you forget the stresses and strains of the day.*

▶ *The good use of hot colours in a room instils cheerfulness and stimulates the senses.*

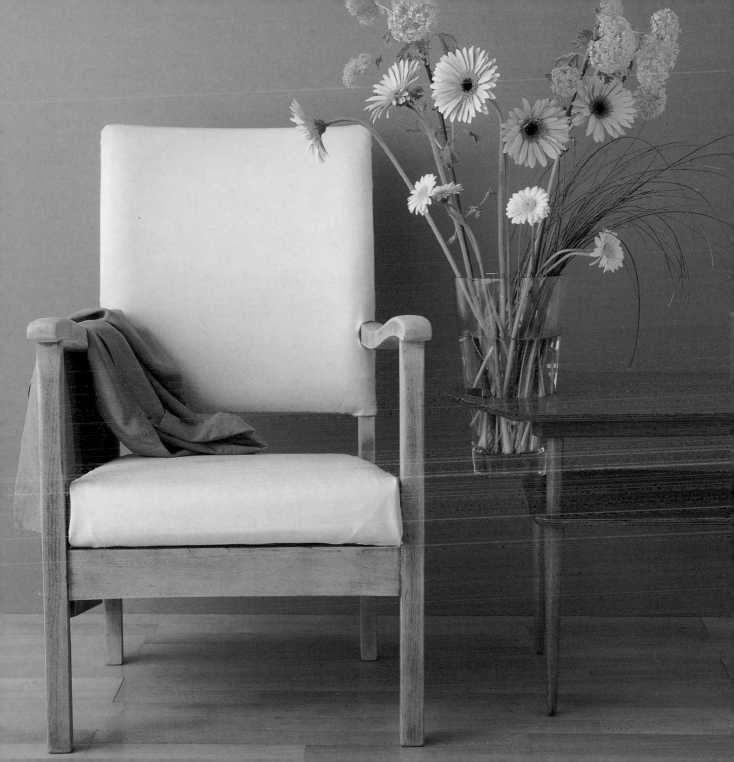

USING INTERIOR DECOR EFFECTIVELY

The physical and psychological effects of colour should be taken into consideration whenever you are decorating your home or office. You can use colour in these areas for therapeutic reasons as well as just visual enjoyment. Blending colours successfully can help to alleviate depression, nervous breakdowns and aggression. In fact, all mental, emotional and physical problems can be alleviated if you understand the language of colour.

When you are deciding how to decorate a room it is important to think about the effects the colours you use will have on its occupants. Consider how the room will be used, but also the people who will use it: do they have any problems that could be alleviated or worsened by your colour choices? What are their ambitions and aims?

Don't forget the furniture, flooring and fabrics that are to be used, and the practicalities of making any colour changes: it is far easier to change the colour of a wall than it is to replace a fitted carpet or expensive furniture.

Take into consideration the size and shape of each room: the stronger the colour, the smaller a room will seem. Small rooms tend to look more spacious decorated in single pale colours. Colours become more intense in larger areas than in small ones, and a strong colour can enclose a room, causing claustrophobia. Dark narrow rooms need light, clear

▼ *Paint your china to introduce beneficial colours to your dining room.*

▼ *Yellow decor in a kitchen inspires efficiency, with no time wasted.*

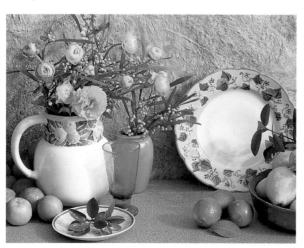

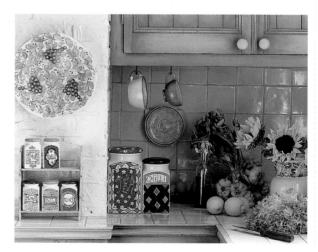

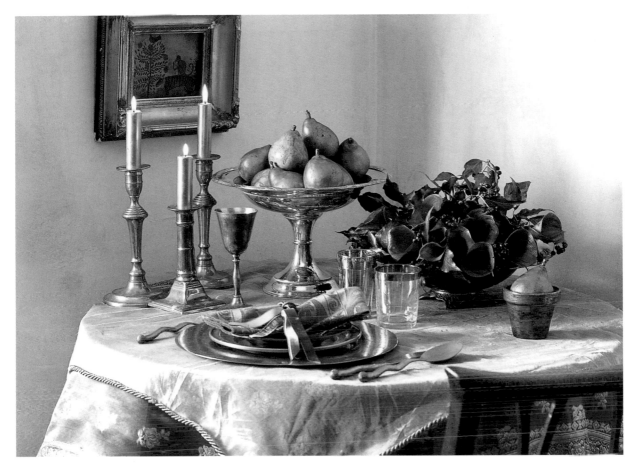

▲ *Use gold accessories in the dining room for a feeling of well-being among your guests.*

colours. You can also alter the apparent shape of a room by the correct use of colour, for example, a darker ceiling shortens high walls, whereas painting the ceiling in a paler colour than the walls opens up a room wonderfully.

Check how much daylight the space gets before using white, as it can be tiring for the eyes and cause frustration. Dark colours in a room may look good with the sun on them, but will become several shades duller at night in artificial light. If you are painting only one wall in a different colour, do not choose a wall where there is a door or window as this dissipates the colour energy.

HOW TO ENHANCE THE MOOD OF YOUR HOME

The colours of your home should be well balanced to suit your needs or purposes, and to minimize stressful problems.

ENTRANCE HALL

A hallway can have a warm, strong colour that is welcoming, such as coral pink, peach or gold. Green in the hall would suggest to guests that you are hospitable and welcoming hosts.

▼ *The complementary colours of red and blue create a harmony in this hall space.*

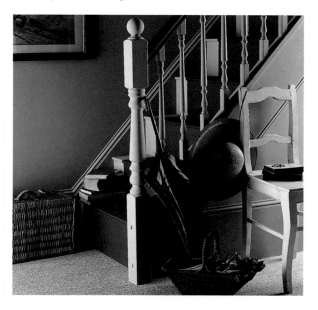

LIVING ROOM

Yellow promotes a feeling of well-being and will put people in a good humour. Brown can give a sense of security. Beige goes anywhere, but you need to introduce one or two stronger colours with it.

DINING ROOM

Orange in a room helps to overcome shyness, but red and orange will make you eat more quickly. Green will help to counteract an overload of red.

KITCHEN

A blue kitchen is inclined to slow you down just when you need to be chopping and peeling energetically. Yellow decor in a kitchen inspires efficiency, with no time wasted.

BEDROOM

Red in a bedroom tends to stimulate too much and cause sleeplessness; indigo would be a better colour to use to avoid insomnia. Indigo in the bedroom is also a useful colour if you suffer from headaches.

BATHROOM

Turquoise is a good colour to choose for your bathroom, where it will feed the nervous system. Add a touch of blue for calmness. Add plants and seashells around the bath, with rich dark green candles for detoxification.

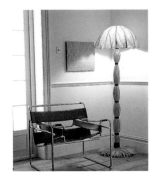

▲ *The earthy brown chair and wooden floor will encourage the sitter to develop their full potential.*

▶ *This blue and white combination helps relaxation and promotes a feeling of safety.*

▼ *Adding the colour red to a kitchen will stimulate action and speed up efficiency*

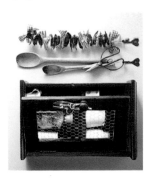

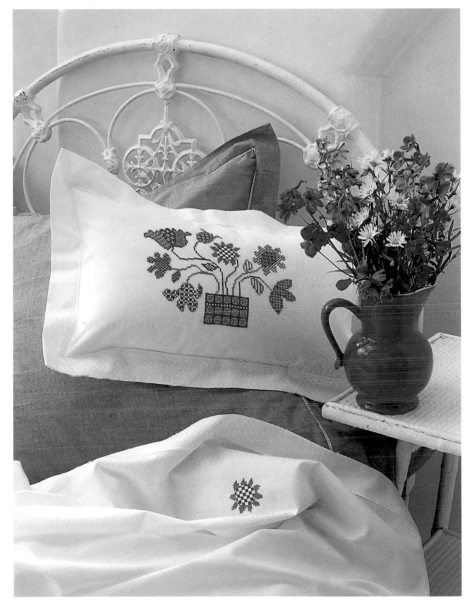

HOW TO ENHANCE THE MOOD OF YOUR OFFICE

A few decades ago, coloured decor for offices was almost unthinkable. Drab browns, grey and dark green were the norm. Today, the trend is to make the most of the effect that colour has on people and the advantages this can create. Promoting the effective use of colour in the office is important both for the comfort of the employees and the productivity of the business. Improperly applied, colour can interfere and distract from work, but it is best to avoid white offices. Brown creates tiredness and non-production; grey induces depression and melancholy; black restricts movement and keeps everything on hold. If

▼ *Incorporate red in your office equipment to boost zest, energy and drive.*

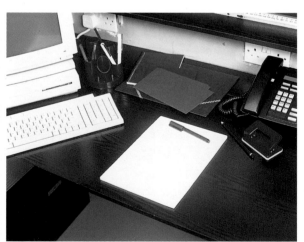

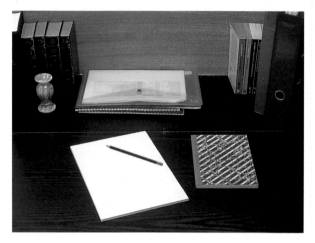

▲ *Blue in the study area will bring a sense of calm and promote inspiration for the writer.*

you use beige, add green or rose to alleviate the negative slackness that too much beige can bring.

Don't forget details like stationery, as they also make a colour statement. You could even consider changing from the standard white, which can cause distraction from the written word. Refer to the psychological meanings of colours to choose the appropriate one for your company's image.

THE CITY OFFICE

Offices in which activity is high, in areas such as sales and banking, should use red upholstery. This definitely puts workers in the hot seat and adds

▲ *Green can be useful in the office when your main aim is to bring abundance and money.*

impetus and drive to their performance. Add green walls to counteract the red and reduce headaches that are brought on by the pressure of work.

THE EXECUTIVE OFFICE

When you are the boss you need an office where employees and directors can talk to you and at the same time be reminded that you lead the way. A rich purple carpet gives an impression of big ideas and creativity along with luxury. Gold decor encourages trust and loyalty, but don't forget to add green plants to represent money and balance.

THE OPEN-PLAN OFFICE

For a large office that is partitioned, you would be well advised to make the overall decor a basic cream and introduce bright colours for the paintwork. Use orange, emerald green, rose and rich blue. If only one colour can be used, choose a bright turquoise as this will enable people to feel a little privacy.

THE HOME OFFICE

An office at home can encourage the workaholic. An effective combination would be a royal blue carpet with yellow curtains and pale blue or primrose yellow walls: this should succeed in keeping the business in the office only, and not allow the work to penetrate into your personal life.

THE WHITE ROOM

It became very fashionable a few years ago to have totally white decor in a room: white carpet, sofa, walls – in fact, the whole apartment was turned over to pristine white. The promotion of white interiors had more to do with enhancing the careers of decorators and designers than with benefiting the occupants.

An overload of perfectionist white, if you are surrounded by it for too long, will cause agitation and frustration. Too much of any colour has its side effects. So it is with white decor. Placing one red object in the room, or arranging flowers of the same hue, will dissipate the barren sterility that too much white can cause.

▼ *Look at all the coloured gels before deciding which colour is right for the way you feel now.*

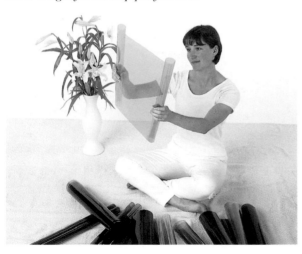

The all-white tradition in hospitals could do with a little breaking up by the introduction of other colours. Lavender would be a good idea for post-operation recovery rooms, blue would help to calm fear and pre-operative nerves, while peach and pink would introduce a little stimulation when it's time to get patients up on their feet again. You can help friends and relatives staying in hospital by taking in appropriately coloured flowers.

The benefit of an all-white room in your own home is that it offers, at the flick of a switch, the perfect healing sanctuary. By installing a lighting system that enables you to turn on any colour at will, you can flood the room with your chosen colour. This enables you to be bathed in a colour treatment for maximum health and well-being. Imagine returning home after a hard day's work in need of some rejuvenation. All you have to do is turn on the red light and sit in the room swamped with a rich, red vibration for 10 minutes.

You can also achieve this effect by acquiring a free-standing spotlight and selecting a coloured slide or gel appropriate to your needs. Place the gel over the spotlight, taking care to ensure it is not touching the hot bulb. Turn off any other lights in the room and turn on the spotlight. Sit in the path of the spotlight's ray and bathe in the coloured light for an instantly available, on-the-spot therapy.

▶ *Bathe yourself in the green vibration to bring in positive thoughts and creativity.*

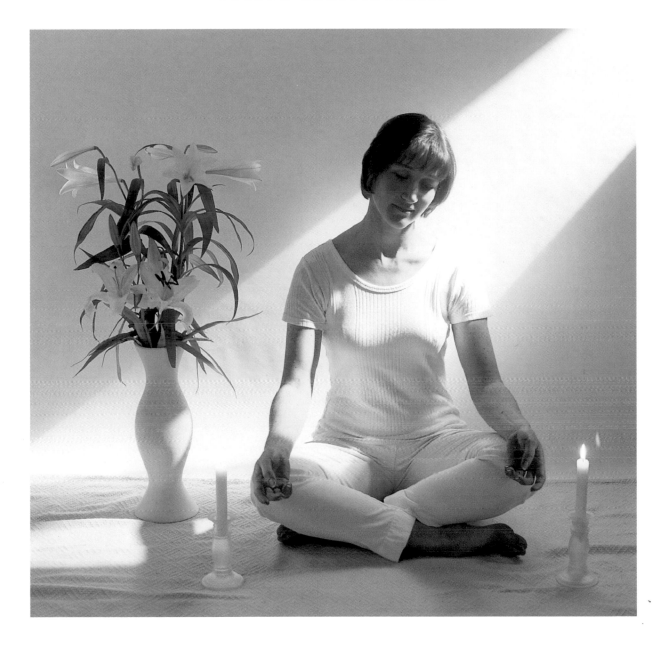

HEALING WITH COLOUR

DISEASE IS REGARDED AS an enemy, but it is possible to think of it as your best friend. It is telling you the truth about yourself, and the ways in which you are out of harmony with the "real" you.

There are several ways of harnessing the vibration of colour for health and well-being. Colour does more than just please the eye. You can eat it, drink it, wear appropriately coloured clothes or jewellery, absorb the colour through your skin or eyes, or decorate and light your home specifically with colour in mind.

Wholesome, fresh food will be full of colour energy. Become aware of the different colours of foods you choose, as your preferences can convey valuable information about yourself via the meanings

◀ *Contemplate with yellow to release yourself from exhaustion and depletion.*

▶ *Learn to colour yourself healthy, wealthy and wise.*

▶ *Focus on a crystal to centre yourself, and to receive divine healing.*

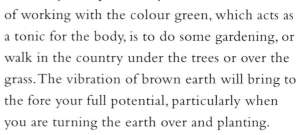

of your chosen colours.

Your home can be a haven of health when you decorate and furnish it in the appropriate colours. House plants are a must. An extremely therapeutic way of working with the colour green, which acts as a tonic for the body, is to do some gardening, or walk in the country under the trees or over the grass. The vibration of brown earth will bring to the fore your full potential, particularly when you are turning the earth over and planting.

Working with colour and understanding the connection between yourself and colour offers a key to good health and vitality.

NOTE
Colour healing can be combined in a complementary way with other therapies. It should not be used as a replacement for medical treatment.

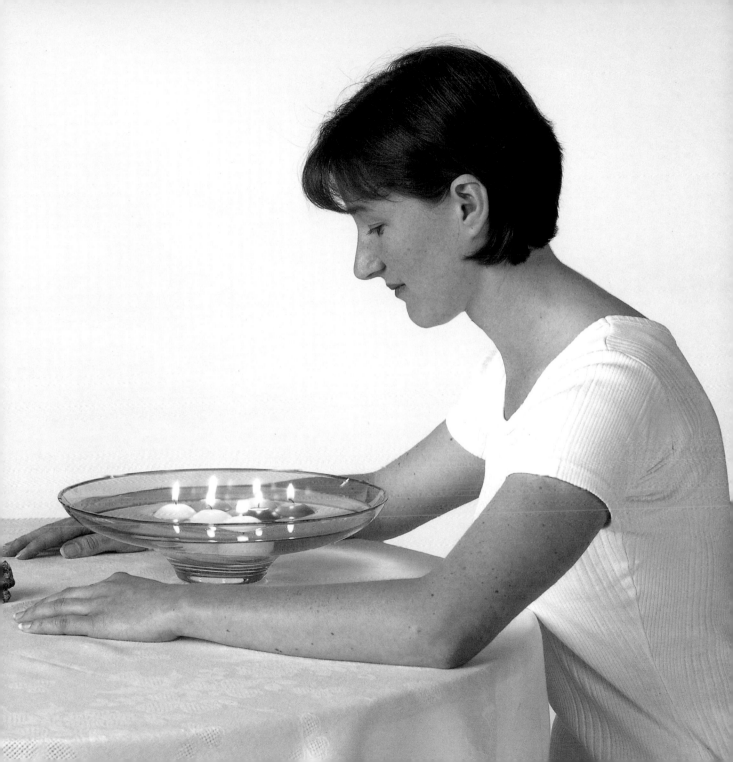

MOOD FOODS

Different coloured foods can be taken in by the body to heal and stimulate health. Eating the appropriate coloured foods can help to rejuvenate and balance the system.

Seek out foods that are organically grown with no additives, as this will keep the colour vibration alive. Processed and junk foods are dead foods. Microwaving food removes its colour energy, and will create internal disharmony.

Red, orange and yellow foods are always hot and stimulating. Green food can be used to balance the body and is a tonic for the system. Blue, indigo and purple foods are soothing and cooling.

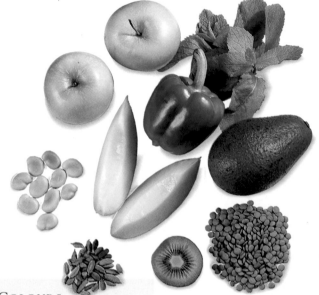

▼ *Red foods promote tireless energy and lively action.*

FOOD COLOURS

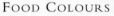

RED: Gives extra energy • Heals lethargy
and tiredness
ORANGE: Creates optimism and change •
Heals grief and disappointment
YELLOW: Encourages laughter, joy and fun •
Heals depression
GREEN: Improves physical stamina •
Heals panic, fear and apprehension
BLUE: Brings peace and relaxation •
Helps concentration • Heals anxiety
INDIGO: Puts back structure into life •
Heals insecurity
PURPLE: Promotes leadership • Heals and
calms the emotionally erratic

▲ *Green foods help prevent self-depletion.*

▼ *Enjoy a rainbow fruit salad to release yourself from colour starvation.*

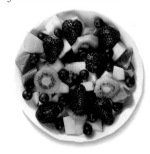

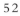

COLOURS FOR DIETING

▶ To encourage weight loss, stimulate your system with the colour yellow. Orange will help the body absorb nutrients from the food.

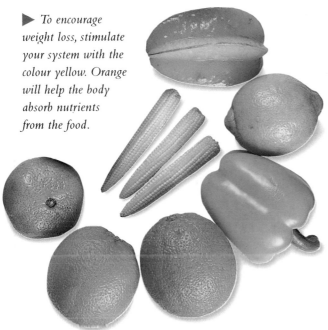

If you are following a sensible diet designed to help you lose or gain weight, the appropriate colour can be used as an aid.

WEIGHT LOSS: YELLOW

To eliminate excess body fat, the colour to use is yellow. Wear it, eat it and drink it. Alternatively, use the Coloured Blooms of Knowledge meditation, visualizing a rich yellow bloom. Psychologically, the colour yellow does not want to carry excess baggage, hence its use in losing weight. Yellow is the nimblest colour of the spectrum and promotes energy and agility both of mind and body. Wear yellow when you exercise and it will keep you moving and pepped up.

WEIGHT GAIN: BLUE

To encourage weight gain, steer yourself towards blue. Wear it, eat it, drink it and visualize it. Blue curbs activity, which allows the calories to gather and turn to flesh. Psychologically, blue does everything quietly and with discretion. It will not be rushed, creating the right emotional environment that is needed if your body is to be given a chance to increase itself. Blue calms the nerves and the glandular system which encourages the curves.

◀ To encourage weight gain, steer yourself towards the blues.

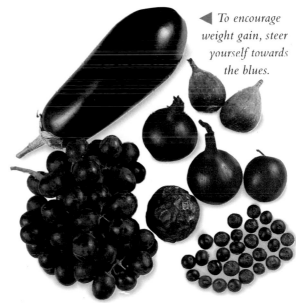

CHROMOTHERAPY

The concept of chromotherapy, or light treatment, is not new. The effect of colour and coloured light has been applied through the ages, from ancient Egyptian temples to the stained glass windows of medieval churches that saturated the congregation with light. Nowadays, paediatricians prescribe a three-day course of blue light for the treatment of jaundice in newborn babies, while modern surgical techniques use laser beams in place of scalpels. Sunlight itself can be used as a cleanser, killing harmful bacteria. Containing all the colours of the spectrum in equal amounts, sunlight is an important nutrient and is vital to our well-being.

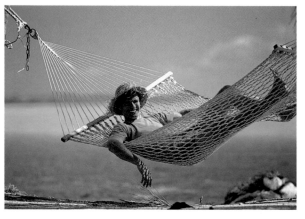

◀ *A moderate amount of sunlight can be used as a cleanser.*

The principle involved in chromotherapy is simple. By using different coloured gels or slides in front of high-powered lamps, you can bathe the body or pinpoint a specific problem area with any colour you require for healing. The application of different coloured lights directed on to the physical form can bring about relief both for the body and the spirit. The recipient of the treatment can either lie down or sit in a chair, with the lamp directed towards them. If in any doubt, and for serious illness, consult a medical practitioner.

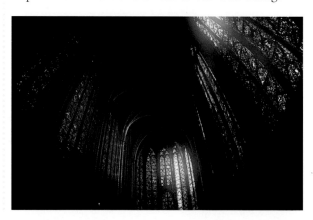

◀ *Sunlight through stained glass is a wonderful way to receive coloured light.*

▶ *Chromotherapy can be used on specific areas: here, the elbow is pinpointed with healing orange to help release stiff ligaments.*

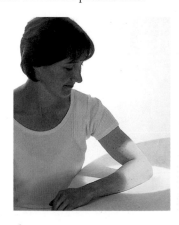

COLOUR HEALING AIDS

The therapeutic power of colour can be applied using a variety of other aids and tools. Check the colour profiles for guidance on the colours to use.

CRYSTALS

Gaze at crystals of many colours, until you become aware of which one beckons to you. The colour connection will give you a key to issues that need addressing. Use the appropriate colour for any ailment, such as blue crystals for a sore throat, or a rose quartz if you need a little comfort or love. Just pop it into your pocket so that you can carry it around. Touch it occasionally, feeling its vibration.

COLOURED CARDS

Colour a set of white cards, shuffle them and set out three cards every day. The first one shows the morning's prospects; the second one lunchtime and the third card represents activities later in the day. If your last card is contractive blue or indigo, you certainly won't be going out that night.

▼ *Wrap yourself in pure colour vibration with turquoise silk to calm the central nervous system.*

CLOTHES

Clothes can be worn to boost any form of healing or to enhance a mood. The skin absorbs very little colour vibration from the material, but psychologically the colour has a profound effect on the person wearing the clothes and also on other people. If you need to wear a colour that you can't stand, then introduce it as underwear in a paler tint, such as peach instead of orange. When colour is paler, the body can absorb it more easily.

By wrapping coloured silk around your body, you can envelope yourself in pure colour vibration. Even a small, green silk square placed behind your head in a chair can relieve tension and pressure.

TORCHES, WATER AND SALT

A torch can be used to beam the appropriate colour on to a pressure point while it is being stimulated. Colouring a Jacuzzi bath, with its underwater lighting, is a wonderful way of combining water with colour vibration. Salt colour-rubs can be used to help invigorate paralysed limbs. Fill a linen bag with sea salt and impregnate it with colour from a spotlight. Then gently massage it over the body.

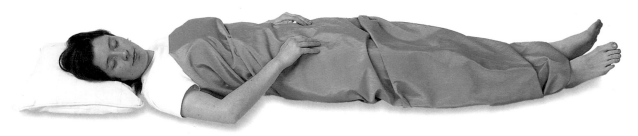

MEDITATION: CELESTIAL HEALING RAYS

Meditating allows you to focus on yourself and gather all those scattered energies. This process, engaging colour as a healing agent, can be performed at any time and anywhere that suits you. You can play forest music if you wish.

1 Close your eyes and envision yourself sitting in a green meadow with a cool, crystal-clear stream running by you, with fragrant flowers all around. The day is clear and bright, with a soft breeze gently swirling around you. The sky is blue, with a scattering of soft, white clouds.

2 Choose a colour that you need for your personal healing and well-being.

▼ *Let the seven colours of the spectrum be your colour guide in meditation.*

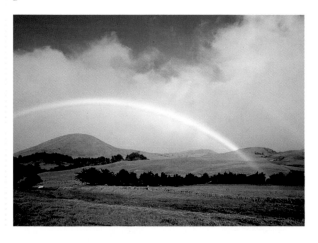

3 Choose one of the clouds in the sky above you. Let this special cloud become filled with your chosen colour and start to shimmer with its coloured, sparkling light.

4 Allow the cloud to float over you; as it does, it will release its coloured shower, allowing a sweet, tinted mist to envelop you as it sparkles all around you. Visualize your chosen colour as stars cascading in all directions.

5 The mist settles on your skin. It gently becomes absorbed through your skin until the colour has entered deep into your very core, completely saturating your system with its healing vibration.

6 Allow the colour to run through your body and bloodstream for at least 3-4 minutes, giving your body a therapeutic rainbow tonic wash.

7 Allow the pores of your skin to open so that the coloured vapour can escape, taking any toxins with it. When the vapour runs clear, you can close your pores.

8 Stay quietly with your cleared, healed body and mind for a few minutes. Take in three deep breaths, releasing each breath gently, before opening your eyes.

▶ *Meditate out of doors to connect to your higher spiritual dimension.*

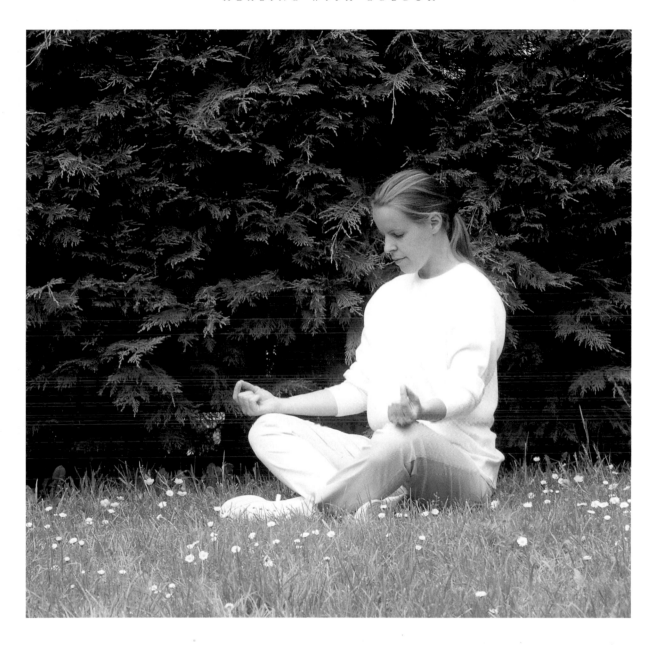

MEDITATION: COLOURED BLOOMS OF KNOWLEDGE

Meditation incorporating colour visualization is thinking in pictures as opposed to words. The colour that emerges gives insight into our emotional state. This meditation allows you to ask for answers to questions that need resolving.

1 Find a comfortable resting-place for yourself and close your eyes.

2 Transport yourself in your mind to an exquisite garden, with you sitting on a grassy mound in the middle of it.

3 There are flowers of every kind and colour surrounding you. Take in the heavenly fragrance while choosing a single blossom.

4 Focus in on the colour of the flower. Ask for guidance with your question while drinking in the colour's vibrations.

5 Let your eyes follow down the green stem into the roots in the earth below.

6 Take a deep breath in and exhale; open your eyes. The colour of the chosen bloom is the key to solving your problem. Let your intuition speak to you, and read the psychological profile of your chosen colour for guidance.

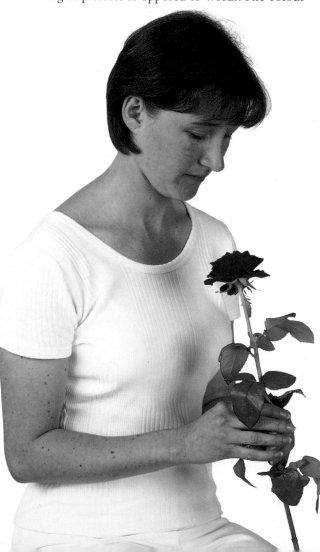

◄ *Red is a colour to rekindle the spirit of physical life.*

MEDITATION: THE GOLDEN CRYSTAL SHOWER

In this meditation the colour gold is used to lift the spirits and encourage the inner light to burn brightly within you.

1 Lying down in a relaxed position, take a deep breath in, and on exhaling imagine yourself lying on a floating sunbed on the ocean or a pool, gently moving with the rhythm of the water.

2 The sky is pale blue and across it is an arch of pure gold. Focus on this shimmering band of sun-gold.

3 After a few moments allow the arch to vibrate gently so that cascades of sparkling golden crystals start to float gently towards you.

4 As they touch your body the crystals turn to golden dew drops that are absorbed by your skin.

5 Feel an internal warmth deep inside you as the golden hue surges around your body, creating a wonderful glow.

6 Take a deep breath in and on exhaling open your eyes. Your mind and body have now been recharged and revitalized.

▶ *Create a breakthrough in your understanding with a burst of sun-gold.*

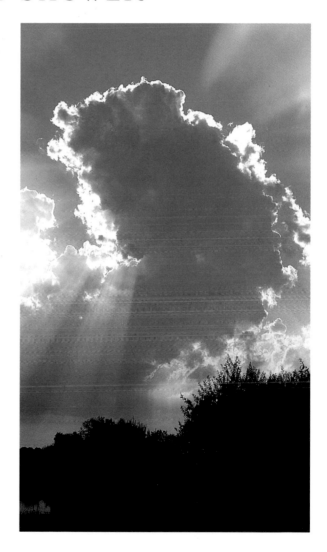

INTUITING COLOUR

Colour is part of your psychic make-up, as inherent as your sight or sense of smell. Psychic ability is a sensitivity we all have to a certain degree – the ability to fine-tune the senses.

The best way to achieve it is simply to make yourself available and clear of mind, so that which is always there can be picked up. It helps to use a colour tool such as a crystal to connect you to the psychic space. Acquiring glimpses into the unseen can give information regarding unanswered questions. Tapping into the intuitive side of yourself means you have access to the whole.

▼ *A simple process using candlelight will enable you to connect to your psychic ability.*

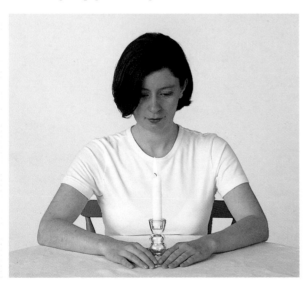

A SIMPLE CANDLELIGHT PROCESS

It is not surprising that mystics are often depicted gazing out towards the light. Without light there is no life. Colour is born from light and as such it can be your guide to infinite truth. To begin using light to develop your psychic sense, focus on the flame of a candle. The candle represents the light force and reminds us that we also glow eternally, as the flame does. This simple candlelight process will enable you to gain access to your psychic colour keys.

1 Light a white candle in a darkened room. Sit directly in front of it.

2 Take a deep breath in and relax, allowing your eyes to focus on the gently flickering flame. Remain in this position for 15 minutes, breathing gently.

3 Close your eyes and you will see colours coming from the dark. Stay with this psychic show of colours until no more appear, or until a bland dullness is present. Remember the colours.

4 Open your eyes, take a deep breath in and exhale. Write down the colour or sequence of colours as they appeared. Practise until you can harness the light easily. The colour parade shown to you will give you answers through your psychic sense.

▶ *Saturate yourself in the calming blue ray to reach a state of peace and tranquility.*

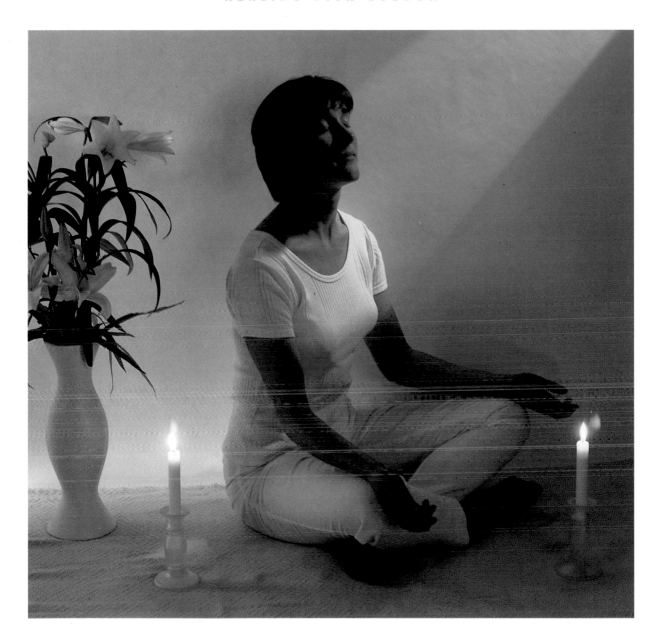

INTUITING COLOUR USING A PENDULUM

Another way to access your intuition is to use a pendulum. A clear crystal one is preferable, but a clear glass bead or button dangling at the end of a piece of chain can do the job quite well.

Begin by tying the crystal or button to the end of a chain or a length of white thread. Hold the other end of the chain between the first finger and thumb so that the crystal hangs down. Place the crystal over the outstretched palm of the other hand and ask the pendulum a question. If it swings round in a circle to the right the answer is "yes". Swinging to the left it is a "no". When the pendulum swings backwards and forwards it is an indication that there is no conclusion.

▶ *Use a pendulum with the colour wheel to materialize information from the unseen.*

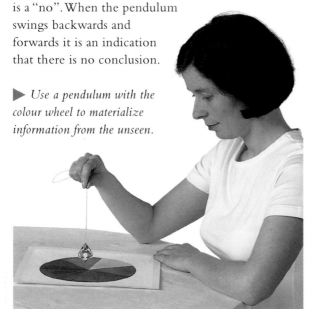

You can use crystals or buttons of different colours for different questions. For instance, if you are seeking information regarding affairs of the heart, use turquoise; for business and finance, use a green crystal.

THE COLOUR WHEEL

Using a large circle of white paper, divide the circle into as many pie-piece wedges as you wish. In each section put a basic colour with its tint and shade: for example red, pink and maroon. You can incorporate as many colours as you wish or fill the whole circle with many shades and tints of one colour only. Hold your pendulum in the centre of the wheel and ask a question. Allow the pendulum to move to whichever section of the board it wants to go to. The colour section it swings towards gives you psychic colour clues to the information you desire. Refer to the psychological profile of your chosen colour to analyse the information.

Always remember that any colour intuiting process can only give indications. The art is in the interpretation. Monitor your findings. You will be surprised at how many of them materialize.

▶ *Transform the rainbow into a colour wheel on paper as a tool to help you gain spiritual insight. Use this page, or create your own wheel including shades and tints of each colour.*

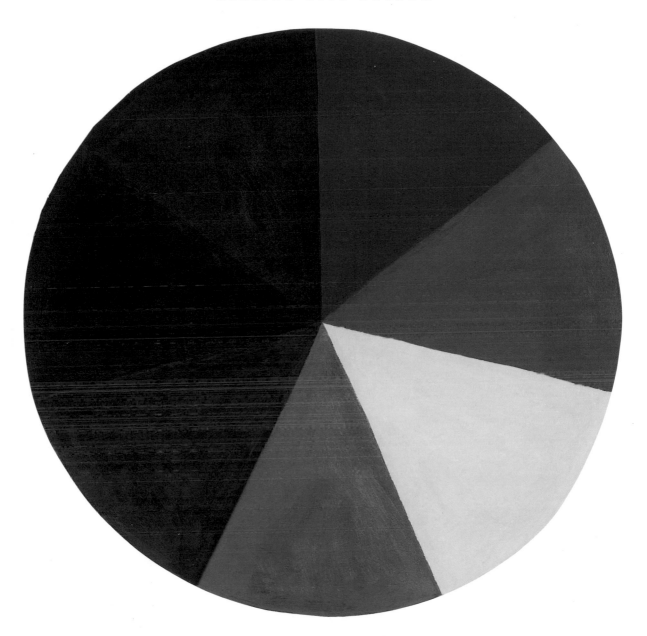

INDEX AND ACKNOWLEDGEMENTS

black, 30
blue, 24-5, 37
brilliance, 14-15

candles, 60
chromotherapy, 54
clothes, 55
colour wheel, 62-3
coloured blooms of knowledge
 meditation, 58
complementary colours, 39
consciousness, colour, 40
crystals, 55

dieting, 53
disease, 50

food, 52-3

gold, 32
golden crystal shower
 meditation, 59
green, 22-3, 37
grey, 35

healing, 50, 55-6
hidden colours, 38
history, 8-9

indigo, 26-7, 37
interior decor, 42-8

intuition, 60-2

light treatment, 54
light waves, 10

meditation, 56-9
moods, enhancing, 44-5

offices, 46-7
orange, 18-19, 37

pendulums, 62
psychic ability, 60
psychology of colour, 12
purple, 28-9, 37

red, 16-17, 36-7

shades, 36-7
silver, 33
spectrum, 10-11

tints, 36-7
turquoise, 34

white, 31
white rooms, 48

yellow, 20-1, 37

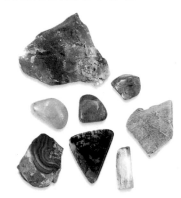

Picture Acknowledgements
The publishers gratefully acknowledge
the following photographers and
photographic agencies for permission
to reproduce their photographs in
this book:
E.T. Archive: 8 (both), 10 (top).
Bruce Coleman Limited: 11, 13,
14 (bottom left), 14 (bottom right),
20 (bottom), 21 (top right), 22 (top),
26 (bottom left), 31 (top), 33 (top),
34 (bottom right), 35 (top right),
54 (bottom left), 56, 59.
Tony Stone Images: 9, 14 (top),
54 (top).

Lilian Verner-Bonds can be
contacted at: Colour Bonds
Association, 137 Hendon Lane,
London N3 3PR. Please enclose a
stamped, self-addressed envelope.